Charles Ross

Major depressive disorder precursors, predictors and coping mechanism

Analysis focused on undergraduate students

GRIN Verlag

Bibliografische Information der Deutschen Nationalbibliothek:

Die Deutsche Bibliothek verzeichnet diese Publikation in der Deutschen National-bibliografie; detaillierte bibliografische Daten sind im Internet über http://dnb.d-nb.de/ abrufbar.

Dieses Werk sowie alle darin enthaltenen einzelnen Beiträge und Abbildungen sind urheberrechtlich geschützt. Jede Verwertung, die nicht ausdrücklich vom Urheberrechtsschutz zugelassen ist, bedarf der vorherigen Zustimmung des Verlages. Das gilt insbesondere für Vervielfältigungen, Bearbeitungen, Übersetzungen, Mikroverfilmungen, Auswertungen durch Datenbanken und für die Einspeicherung und Verarbeitung in elektronische Systeme. Alle Rechte, auch die des auszugsweisen Nachdrucks, der fotomechanischen Wiedergabe (einschließlich Mikrokopie) sowie der Auswertung durch Datenbanken oder ähnliche Einrichtungen, vorbehalten.

Imprint:

Copyright © 2011 GRIN Verlag GmbH
Druck und Bindung: Books on Demand GmbH, Norderstedt Germany
ISBN: 978-3-656-61075-5

This book at GRIN:

http://www.grin.com/en/e-book/269790/major-depressive-disorder-precursors-pre-dictors-and-coping-mechanism

GRIN - Your knowledge has value

Der GRIN Verlag publiziert seit 1998 wissenschaftliche Arbeiten von Studenten, Hochschullehrern und anderen Akademikern als eBook und gedrucktes Buch. Die Verlagswebsite www.grin.com ist die ideale Plattform zur Veröffentlichung von Hausarbeiten, Abschlussarbeiten, wissenschaftlichen Aufsätzen, Dissertationen und Fachbüchern.

Visit us on the internet:

http://www.grin.com/

http://www.facebook.com/grincom

http://www.twitter.com/grin_com

Major Depressive Disorder: Precursors, Predictors, and Coping Mechanism among

Undergraduate Students

Major Depressive Disorder: Precursors, Predictors, and Coping Mechanism among Undergraduate Students

1. Preface

Major Depressive Disorders is one of the first disorders to be recognized among humanity. A number of psychologists and psychiatrists have come up with theories and myths that explain the origin of MDD. Ancient Egyptians identified the brain to be the body organ that was in charge of human consciousness (James Herbert, 2009). They believed that brain disorders could be caused by both supernatural factors and also other factors that were within human control. The Old Testament is also one of the earliest evidence of MDD. Examined as literary description of human behavior and society, MDD is described by King David and other author. It is defined as another form of psychological distress. In the earlier days, symptoms associated with MDD as per today's standards include insomnia, fatigue, sadness and fearfulness. It is quite evident that even in the pre-classical period people had acknowledged conditions similar to MDD (James Herbert, 2009). However, the earliest written record of a medical diagnostic condition similar to MDD was in the classical era. It is the melancholia described by the Hippocrates. Melancholia is a sub set of Major Depressive Disorder but in earlier cases the word melancholia was used in place of MDD. In other parts of the world, melancholia is still used to mean MDD in today's diagnostics (Seth Disner, 2011).

Melancholia is an etiological conceptualization of the Hippocrates' time that revolves around the philosophy of the four humors. They believed that human moods, behaviors and emotions were affected by the interaction of the four bodily fluids. These are yellow bile, blood, phlegm

2

and black bile. According to Galen, a Roman physician, individuals' personalities were defined

by the mixing of these four fluids. Based on this framework pathology was thought to arise in

cases of imbalance in the mixing of the fluids. In Greek, melancholia means black bile; as such,

melancholia was believed to arise in cases of overabundance of black bile (Seth Disner, 2011).

Most societies no longer believe in melancholia but the symptoms associated with it are exhibited

in persons suffering from MDD today. Symptoms of melancholia included loss of appetite,

intense continuous pain, insomnia, and diminished interest in formerly pleasurable activities,

difficulty in concentrating, suicidal ideation, irritability, excessive guilt and fatigue (Fishman,

2011).

2. Introduction

MDD is widely distributed among the different age groups and it is a common disorder. Seth

Disner et al (2011) defines MDD as the existence of five or more depressive symptoms; namely

sad mood, fatigue, inability to concentrate, self criticism and suicidal innuendos. It is mental

disorder that generally affects the normal functioning of an individual; the condition affects the

patient's family, school life, and work, eating and sleeping habits (Fishman, 2011). The diagnosis

of MDD is based on mental status examination and proclamations by friends, relatives and the

patients themselves. There are also laboratory tests that could be performed to establish the extent

to which the patient has been affected. Patients are usually treated using antidepressant,

psychotherapy and counseling (Seth Disner, 2011). There has been a rise in the number of

undergraduate students suffering from MDD. This disorder is associated with impairment and

increase in mortality rates. It has grown into a public health problem as it was formerly

overlooked and not much attention was put into treating depressive disorders.

MDD greatly affects the performance and school experience of students. For example, students suffering from depressions are at a higher risk of failing in exams, contemplating suicide or even interpersonal difficulties. Therefore, it is important that programs are put in place to help students with depression. School counselors can play a huge role in implementing programs that help reduce the risk of students getting into depression. MDD is a condition that needs to be actively addressed in colleges and learning institutions (Fishman, 2011). The most recent statistics show that 100 students out of 1000 in an institution are at the risk of experiencing severe depression. People who suffer from depression contract the condition early in life. Depression affects adolescents' thoughts, moods, actions and physical health. If untreated the condition could lead to more severe conditions later in life, could as well lead to early death (Kadison, 2004).

2.1. Research objectives

The purpose of this research is to investigate and analyze the impact of a combination of precursors: predictors of MDD cognitive functioning, interpersonal relationships (peers and family), and substance abuse, self-efficacy and maladaptive coping mechanism (avoidance coping) among a national sample of U.S college students (Schwartz, 2002). It aims at presenting current information on major depressive disorder and coping mechanisms. It is important that the high risk population be taught on the signs and symptoms of this condition. When the people have enough information they are able to seek medication early enough before the condition becomes worse. Research shows that undergraduate students have exhibited an increase in those suffering from MDD (Seth Disner, 2011). This is shown by the increased number of teenage suicide cases in learning institution. The longer the duration which one suffers from MDD the higher the chances of them committing suicide.

Major Depressive Disorder

2.2. Scope of research

This topic of study has been chosen for a number of reasons. The various journals and reports covered here revolve around MDD as a whole. People should be able to identify MDD symptoms early enough. School counselors too need to get the most current information on MDD; this enables them to upgrade the way in which they handle the students. Counselors can look for better mechanisms of helping the students recovering from minor depressions. Early detection of stress and accurate assessment of the condition are one of the most effective mechanisms of preventing depressive disorders (Fishman, 2011)).

Other literatures cover the potential negative effects of MDD. Given its potential negative side effects, it is important that coping mechanism be addressed. Schools should be able to provide prompt referrals for treatment, appropriate treatment and preventive interventions. Early identification is very vital in handling depressive disorder. The more the delay in identifying and treating a depressive condition the worse the situation becomes. Collaboration between school counselors and health professionals can help reduce case of MDD in institutions. This helps reduce the number of students that commit suicide. In multicultural institutions such as colleges, stress is also associated with other conditions such as alcoholism and absenteeism (Fishman, 2011).

Despite the many research works done on the same, very few have completely laid out the symptoms of the condition. Depression among school going students usually goes undetected and untreated. They are often referred and treated for symptoms other than the depression; in some cases they receive inadequate treatment. Caretakers such as parents, teachers, counselors and peers may not be able to tell the difference between a depressed student and one who is just moody. The psychological, hormonal, physical and behavioral changes in school going undergraduates make it difficult to identify MDD early enough (Beverley Haarhoff, 2011). Some health professionals may also in miss the signs of depression since they lack sufficient information on the precursors, predictors and coping mechanisms. Many custodians, parents and school counselors tend to believe that depression is a problem that people grow out of. In most cases, students do not grow out of depression and this develops to MDD. Teachers and parents are also not prepared to prepare depressive symptoms (Fishman, 2011).

2.3.   Structure of the dissertation

This chapter comprises of 6 main parts.

- The first topic provides an introduction to the situation of the Major Depressive Disorders among undergraduate students. It also highlights why this study needs to be conducted. The possible potential positive social changes are also given in the study.

- The second part covers the background of the study; this summarizes the research literature relating to the scope of the dissertation. It also describes the gap in knowledge between the various disciplines of study. This topic is concluded by giving the reason why the study is necessary.

- The third part is the problem statement. This gives a summary of evidence of consensus that the problem is current, relevant and significant to the discipline. This section also frames the problem in a way that builds upon or counters previous research findings focusing primarily on research conducted in the past five years. It also further defines a meaningful gap that exists in the current research literature.

- The fourth section covers the purpose of the study. It provides statement that connects the problem being addressed and the focus of the study. It gives the study intent and quantifies the study.

- The fifth section is the research questions and hypothesis. This gives the research questions and states the null and alternative hypothesis. It gives the theoretical framework of the precursors, predictors and coping mechanisms with regard to Major Depressive Disorders.

- The sixth section is the nature of the study. Here a provision for a concise rationale for selection of the research design is given. This section also covers the methodology used; how the data was collected and from whom.

- The research references and appendices will be listed in the final part of the study.

These are the major parts of the papers, after which such minor sections as conclusion and discussion. There is also definition of the words used and their applicability in the research work.

3. Background of the study

Major Depressive is increasingly becoming a public health issue. Most college students are being affected by this disorder. Carlos et al (2010) reveals that this condition is chronic and recurrent in nature. It is associated with the increased levels of mortality among college going students. Studies currently shows that 100 out of every 1000 college going students experience severe depression at one time in their lives. Depressed students tend to have a low self esteem and think poorly of themselves. It is no wonder, they attempt suicide. There has been a dramatic increase in suicide rates among school going teenagers (Carlos Zalaquett, 2010).

3.1.   Developmental model of depression

Aaron Beck (2008) attempts to integrate the psychological components of a depression; what he also refer to as a cognitive model of depression. Based on his research the only evidence available for depression was negativity in the patient's system. This was shown by the patients self report. Variables accountable for depression included hopelessness, self criticism, suicidal thoughts, Loss of motivation, seclusion and disassociation. The next level of the model was systematic cognitive bias. This involved one concentrating only on the negative aspects of experiences, negative interpretation and blocking of positive thoughts. A question raised during this research was that what factors were responsible for the negative thoughts (Aaron Beck, 2008). Dysfunctional attitudes were identified as the cause of the negativity. A collective number of studies have shown that dysfunctional attitudes and beliefs has been a contribution to depression for many patients. Dysfunctional attitudes are measured using the Dysfunctional Attitudes Scale. These attitudes originate from cognitive structures also known as schemas.

The energy in the schemas varies depending on the intensity of the negative memories and the successive stressful events. When the schemas are activated by the occurrence of a number of recurrent stressful events it translates to negative stimuli and interpretation. The overall negative perception of experiences is what leads to depression. Seth Disnar et al (2011), further notes that the negative perceptions can be shown by sadness, social withdrawal, loss of motivation and hopelessness. The cognitive model was a representation of the factors that support depression; it also forms a framework for developing cognitive therapy (James Herbert, 2009).

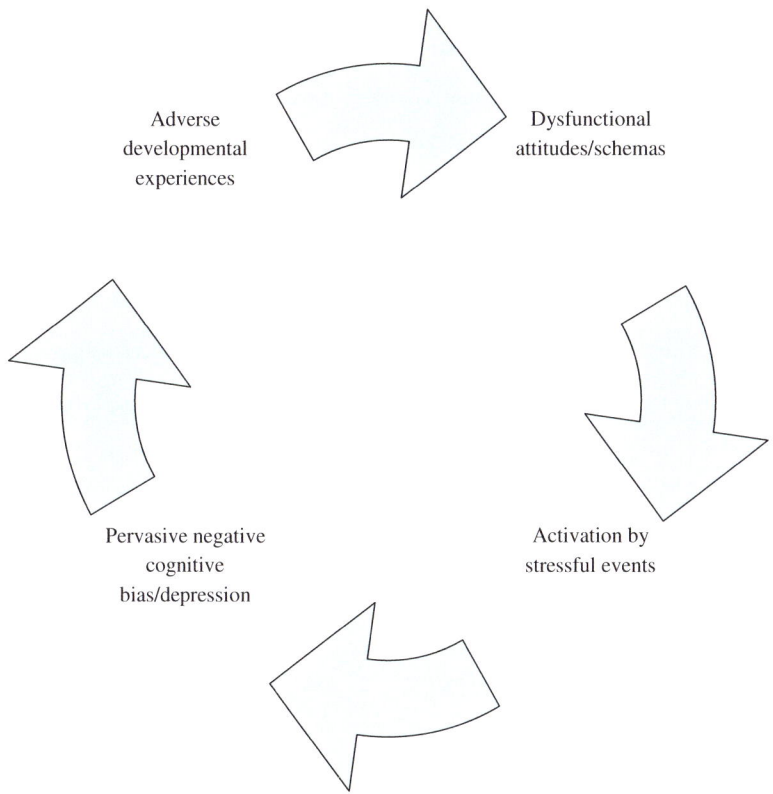

Figure 1: Showing the developmental model of depression (Beck, 2008)

3.2.   Factors contributing to MDD among college going students

Other than the fact that persons between 18 and 24 years are more prone to manifest mental disorders, there are other factors that directly contribute to the increasing number of undergraduates who suffer from MDD. Most undergraduates are within the above stated age range. The academic pressure has also led to students suffering from depression and anxiety (Flatt, 2013). According to a survey conducted by the American College Health Association most students who had suffered from stress cited stress from their school work as a cause of the stress. The students feel pressured to perform well and achieve high grades. Another study conducted by Furr et al (2001) on 1455 students from American University also reveals the same. 53 % of these students cited academic problems to be the leading cause of depression. They began to experience the stress ones they joined the university. High grade expectations form parents and stakeholders make students strive to perform even beyond their abilities. The gap between the reality of how the students perform and how the lecturers and parents expect them to perform is what lead to academic pressures (Furr, 2011).

Watkins et al (2001) also conducted another survey of school counselors to ascertain what could have been the cause of the rising depression among students. Research findings showed that students became nervous as they were not sure if they could obtain what their parents expected them to get. The greatest concern represented by millennial students was college grades and admission. This is alongside the nuclear war, violence and HIV/AIDS pandemic. The research also showed that students who came from small families even experienced more pressure in the need to perform well. The parents focused on them more compared to students who came from large families (Watkins, 2001).

Major Depressive Disorder

Some researchers have identified the increasingly competitive economic environment to be one of the causes for stress among college students (Beverly Haarhoff, 2011). Johnson & Diaz (2011) identifies such pressures as employment conditions as a contributing factor to academic pressure. As soon as undergraduates complete their course they expect to get well paying jobs in the various industries. The job opportunities are few. One has to be extremely smart to obtain a position in the industry. Undergraduates stress on the ability to match up to the job market demands. There has been an increased level of academic competition among undergraduate sand graduates. Students are even forced to study multiple courses at the same time. Other struggle so hard to register for further courses ones they done. The financial resources may not be readily available for one to further their education (Beverly Haarhoff, 2011).

Financial burdens have been cited by many studies as a contributing factor to mental stress among undergraduates (Watkins et al, 2011, Kadison, 2004, Waddel et al, 2002). The cost of learning and interest on students loans have grown high these days. The burden is intolerable by some students especially those from financially less fortunate families. According to a study by Schwartz & Finnie (2002), it was noted that the Canadian higher education had undergone a huge shift as most of the students fee was paid by the students while the government paid just a small amount. Between the year 1989 and 2009, government funding in Canada fell to 55% from 72%. The tuition fee has always been on rise in many economies (Flatt, 2013). Research shows that students who have high debt on student loans are more likely to suffer depressive conditions. Students' perception on debt has a huge effect on their academic performance. The mental health crisis is also heightened by school counselors and health centers that are not prepared to deal with this condition when they arise. There is no health support for students who suffer from depressive disorder. Studies that institution with support service for students who are depressed can only support mild forms of depression (Flatt, 2013).

According to studies by Aaron Beck (2008), cognitive vulnerability originates from ones childhood. For instance, when one loses a loved one at a young age they are more inclined to suffer from depressive disorder in the future. Individuals with dysfunctional attitudes are more vulnerable to recurrence of a depression; with time the condition might become worse (Beck, 2008). This research expressed the cognitive reactivity concept, which illustrated that stress was caused by fluctuation of a patient's negative attitudes due to the daily events. Cognitive reactivity has been illustrated using clinical experiments and priming interventions such as social rejection film clip, contrived failure, sad music and imaging of sad autobiographical memories among others. Symptoms of depression need not be attributed to substances, death of loved ones or medical conditions. In relation to Beck's model of depression, each component is believed to maintain a given depressive event. This is against speculations that only some parts of the model are directly related to the causal events (Beck, 2008).

Seth Disner et al (2011), furthers Beck's research by establishing the correlates to the model of depression. This study also reviews the structural and neurobiological factors associated with depression.

Major Depressive Disorder

Works Cited

Beck, A. (2008). *The evolution of the Cognitive Model of depression and its neurobiological*

correlates. ajp.psychiatryonline.org: Am J Psychiatry.

Beverly Haarhoff, R. F. (2011*). Evaluating the content and Quality of Cognitive Behavioural*

Therapy case conceptualizations. New Zealand Journal of Psychology *, Vol. 40* (Issue No.

3), 104-115.

Carlos Zalaquett, A. S. (2010). *Major Depression and dysthymic disorder in adolescents*

The critical role of school counselors. University of South Florida: Vistas.

Flatt, A. K. (2013, Winter). *College Quarterly.* Retrieved October 12, 2013, from *A Suffering*

generation: Six factors contributing to the men tal health of crisis in North American

higher education: http://www.senecac.on.ca/quarterly/2013-vol16-num01-

winter/flatt.html

Furr, R. S., Westfield, S. J., McConnell, N. G., & Jenkins, M. J. (2001). *Suicide and depression among college students: A decade later*. Professional Psychology: Research and Practice, 32, 97-100.

James Herbert, B. G. (2009). *The importance of Theory in Cognitive Behaviour Therapy*. Philadelphia: Drexel University.

Kadison, R. D., & DeGeronimo, T. F. (2004).*College of the overwhelmed: The campus mental health crisis and what to do about it* (pp. 58-60). San Francisco, CA: Jossey-Bass.

Schwartz, S. Finnie. R. (2002*). Student loans in Canada: An analysis of borrowing and repayment*. Economics of Education Review. 21, 497-512.

Seth Disner, C. B. (2011). *Neural Mechanisms of the cognitive model of depression.*

Philadelphia: Macmillan Publishers.

Watkins, D. C., Hunt, J., & Eisenberg, D. (2011*). Increased demand for mental health services on college campuses: Perspectives from administrators*. Qualitative Social Work, *11*(3), 319-337.

Waddell C., Offord R., Shepherd A. (2002). *Child psychiatric epidemiology and Canadian public policy-making: the state of the science and the art of the possible*. Canadian Psychiatry, 47(9), 825– 832.